My Mom's Having a Baby

My Mom's Having a Baby

By Elaine Evans Rushnell

Illustrated with drawings and photographs from the teleplay

Based on the Emmy-Award-winning "ABC Afterschool Specials" Program

Created by Elaine Evans Rushnell and Susan Fichter Kennedy

Produced by DePatie-Freleng Enterprises, Inc.

GROSSET & DUNLAP
A FILMWAYS COMPANY
Publishers · New York

MY MOM'S HAVING A BABY, based on the Emmy-Award-Winning
"ABC Afterschool Specials" Program, created by Elaine Evans Rushnell
and Susan Fichter Kennedy, produced by DePatie-Freleng
Enterprises, Inc., and broadcast by ABC Television Network

Text copyright © 1978 by Elaine Evans Rushnell
Illustrations and photographs on pp. 9-23, 25-32, 37-40,
41 (top), 42-45, 46 (bottom), 47-52, 54, 56 (top), 61, 64
copyright © 1978 by DePatie-Freleng Enterprises, Inc.
Photographs on cover and pp. 24, 34-36, 41 (bottom), 46 (top),
53, 55, 56 (bottom), 57-60 copyright © 1977 by American
Broadcasting Companies, Inc.

Library of Congress Catalog Card Number: 77-95422
ISBN: 0-448-16057-9 (Trade Edition)
ISBN: 0-448-13486-1 (Library Edition)
Published simultaneously in Canada
Printed in the United States of America

For Robin and Hilary

Petey Evans woke up and lay staring at the ceiling for a long time. Gradually, his gaze wandered around the room, taking in every detail. The light-blue walls were decorated with all of his favorite treasures—posters, pennants, souvenirs, certificates, a shrunken head, snapshots—lots of interesting things that his mother lumped into one category . . . clutter. Over the bed, his red baseball hat hung on a big hook. The hat was his number-one treasure. He reached for it and put it on, then plopped back down to study the room some more.

Ordinarily, he didn't pay that much attention to his room, but today was different. This room was never going to be the same again. Nothing was ever going to be the same again, just because his mom was going to have a baby.

And Petey was going to have a roommate.

Baby roommates involved making lots of changes besides the diaper kind. His dad was going to repaint the walls, move the furniture around, and bring in a crib and a changing table. Petey wished they lived in a bigger house, maybe one with about twelve bedrooms.

Petey's dad rapped on the door and walked in. "Time to get up, sport," he said. "We've got a lot to do today, and I want to get started."

Petey kicked the covers off and looked at his bare feet. "Okay, Dad, I'll be right down."

Mr. Evans leaned against the doorway and looked around at Petey's clutter collection. "You know, I'll have to take all this stuff off the walls when I paint."

Petey concentrated on the big toe on his right foot. It looked longer than the big toe on his left foot. He really didn't want to hear all the details of how his dad was going to wreck his room.

"Pete?"

"Huh?"

"I said you can put it all back as soon as the paint dries. The baby's not going to care."

Petey sat up as his dad left and breathed a big sigh of relief. At least it wouldn't look like a regular nursery. Nobody hangs a shrunken head in a nursery.

He got dressed and straightened his bed covers, then put his hat back on and grabbed his baseball mitt.

He was glad it was Saturday. That meant a ball game right after breakfast. He ran down the hall and skidded to a halt at the top of the stairs. He sat on the top step and slid down the whole flight on the seat of his pants.

Bumpety, thump, thump, thump. "Ouch!" It would have been a neat ride if he hadn't bitten his tongue.

In the kitchen, Mr. and Mrs. Evans were sitting at the table. Mrs. Evans glanced up and smiled. She was so pretty. Fat, but pretty.

"Hurt yourself, Petey?" she asked. "Why don't you try *walking* down the stairs for a change?"

Petey sat down, drank his juice, and looked into his cereal bowl, puzzled. "I'll make a deal with you, Mom," he said. "I'll try walking down the stairs if you'll tell me what this is in my bowl."

"It's Whammo Flakes," she answered. "I bought it because it has ten different vitamins in it. At least try it."

"Hold it, Pete," Mr. Evans said. "No hats at the table. Once in a while we like to see the top of your head."

Petey shrugged and flipped his hat onto the counter. Mrs. Evans handed Petey a spoon and poured milk on the Whammo Flakes. They wilted instantly. Petey squinted and put a spoonful into his mouth. Yu-uck. They tasted like wet sawdust.

"Mom," he said. "Your doctor said you need to take vitamins. I'm not going to have a baby. Why can't I have rice krispies or something?"

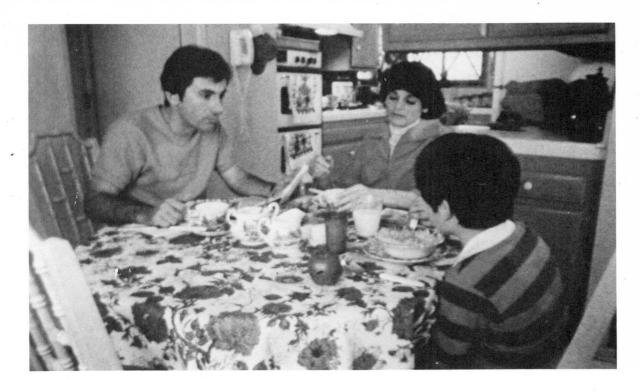

Mrs. Evans said, "I just thought you'd like something different for a change. They can't be that bad."
She dipped her spoon into the bowl and helped herself to a big mouthful. Petey watched her. Mr. Evans watched her too. Mrs. Evans was chewing and swallowing, and she had a funny expression on her face.

Finally Mr. Evans said, "Well?"

She swallowed again and said, "They really have a very unusual flavor . . . sort of like. . . ."

"Sawdust," Petey interrupted.

"Exactly!" Mrs. Evans said. "Petey, why don't you have a nice bowl of rice krispies while I figure out what I'm going to do with a king-size box of vitamin-packed sawdust."

Petey fixed himself another bowl of cereal and stood at the counter, eating it. He looked at his mom. She was upset about the Whammo Flakes. She got upset about all kinds of little things lately. She was always saying "Ohh, Jim," or "Oh, Petey," as though everything were hopeless. Today she was upset because they'd waited until now to redecorate Petey's room.

"Ohh, Jim," she said. "Why do I always let things go until the last minute? The doctor said the baby's due any day now, and. . . . Oh, Petey, speaking of doctors, you have an appointment with Dr. Smith for your checkup on Monday. Remind me. Okay?"

"Okay, Mom," Petey said. "I won't forget."

Mr. Evans patted her hand. "Don't worry, hon," he said. "Everything's going to be just fine."

Petey set his dish in the sink and put his hat back on. He grabbed his mitt and went out the door. "I've got to go or they're going to start without me," he said.

Mr. Evans followed Petey. "Make sure you're home by noon," he said. "I want you to clean out your closet."

"It is clean," Petey said.

"Pete, it's a mess. You can throw out all those broken toys and put the rest in boxes."

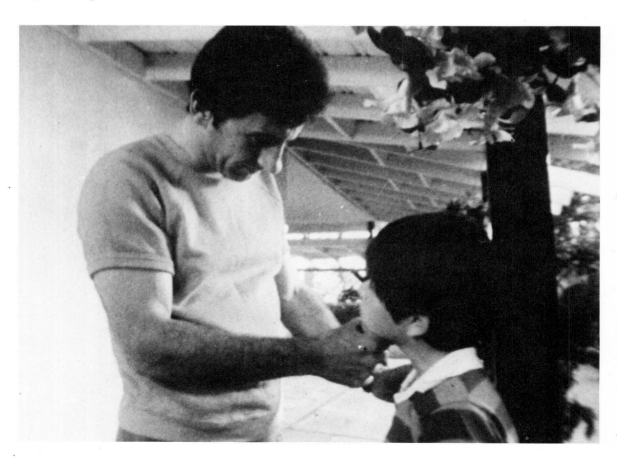

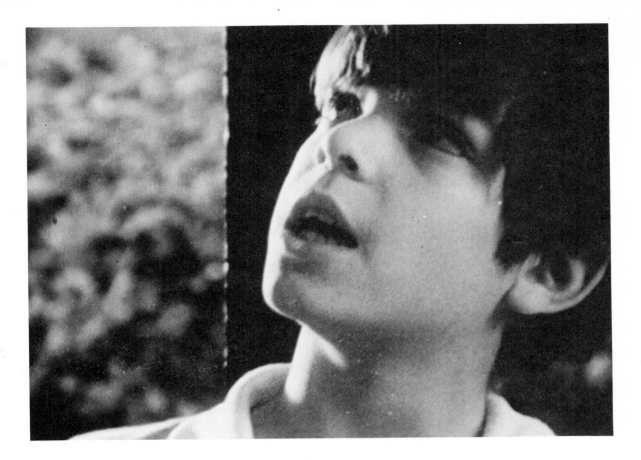

"*Okay*, okay, Dad, I get the message."

Mr. Evans went inside, letting the screen door slam behind him, and Petey heard his mother say "Ohh, Jim" in her hopeless voice. He cut across the lawn, punching his mitt and looking down at the grass.

"Petey!"

The voice behind him was loud and shrill and unmistakably Kelly Driscoll's.

"Oh, brother," Petey mumbled in *his* hopeless voice. First the Whammo Flakes, and now Kelly. He kept walking.

"Hey, Pete, wait up!"

That was Oscar, his best friend, so Petey turned around. Kelly was flying down the sidewalk, her long hair swinging around her face. Oscar was running, trying to keep up with her.

11

"Honestly, Pete, didn't you hear me call you?" Kelly tossed her hair and stood with her hands on her hips.

"Kel, I could hear you if you were calling me from the next town."

"Touchy, touchy," she chided.

Oscar was out of breath and looked like a walking sporting-goods store. He was carrying two baseball bats, a catcher's mitt, chest guard, and face mask.

Petey reached for the bats and the chest guard.

Oscar huffed and puffed. "We flipped a coin to see who was going to carry the stuff, and I lost." Oscar always lost; Kelly always flipped the coin.

She really was a pain most of the time. She could also outpitch anyone else on the team. She was what Petey's dad called a necessary evil. But Petey and Oscar were used to her. They'd all been friends for years, and every so often Kelly surprised them and acted normal.

"What are you so uptight about?" she asked. "Afraid we're going to lose the game?" She didn't wait for Petey to answer. "I'm pitching, so it'll be a piece of cake."

Petey and Oscar rolled their eyes and groaned.

The game wasn't exactly a piece of cake, even though Kelly's pitching arm was in great shape.

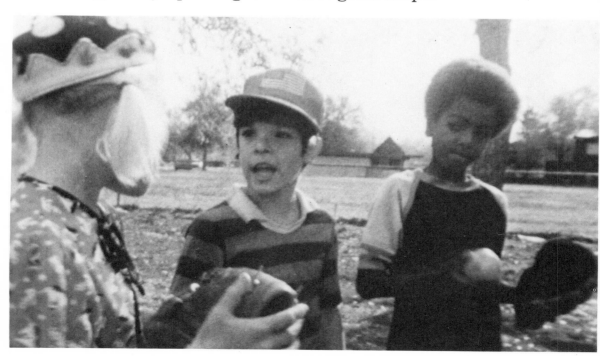

Unfortunately, so was her mouth.

They'd won, but Petey was so annoyed with Kelly it was hard to be happy about the game.

"Why do you always do that?" he asked her.

"Do what?"

"Try to run the whole game. I nearly fell over when you started to explain the rules to the Umpire!!"

"Well," she said, "it looked like a bad call to me. I just wanted to make sure he knew what he was doing."

Petey slapped his forehead in disbelief. "You're un-real, Kel."

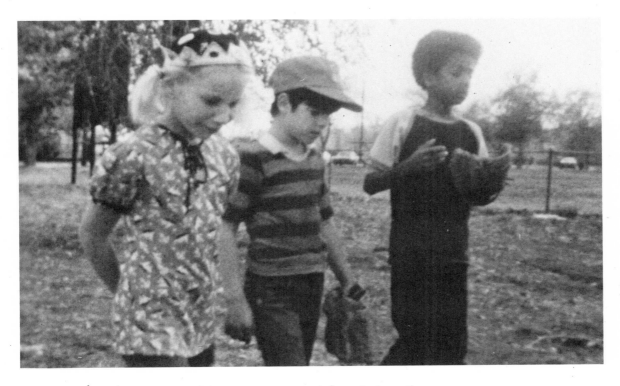

"Look, we won the game, so quit griping."
She didn't like being pushed. The umpire had already given her a piece of his mind.

Oscar wasn't paying any attention to their bickering. He was preoccupied with blowing a bubble.

He felt about bubble gum the way Petey felt about his red hat. Right now he was working on a bubble that was almost as big as his face. They were the best kind, because when they got that big you could see right through them and everything looked pink.

Splat!!

Petey and Kelly turned just as the bubble burst and deflated, covering Oscar's face.

Petey loved it when Oscar did that. He collapsed on the ground and rolled over, laughing.

Kelly groaned. "Honestly, Oscar, you look like your face is melting." She gave Oscar one of her withering glances and sat down next to Petey.

Oscar dropped to his knees and busied himself with pulling the gum off.

The three of them lay flat on their backs, looking up at the sky. Big puffy clouds rolled by like gobs of cotton.

Oscar propped himself up on one elbow and turned to Petey. "Are you going to play this afternoon?"

Petey sat up. "Naw, I've got to help my dad get the room ready for the baby."

"When is your mother going to have that baby?" Kelly asked. "She sure is big."

"I don't know," Petey answered. "Pretty soon, I guess." He stood up and started to walk away.

"Where ya going?" Oscar called, scrambling to catch up.

Kelly jumped to her feet and joined them. "Petey has to go home and fold diapers." she chanted.

"Lay off, Kel," Petey warned.

"Touchy, touchy, touchy," she went on. "I think it's neat your mom's having a baby. I'm the baby in my family, and I'm fantastic!" She shrieked with delight and ran down the sidewalk. Petey and Oscar took

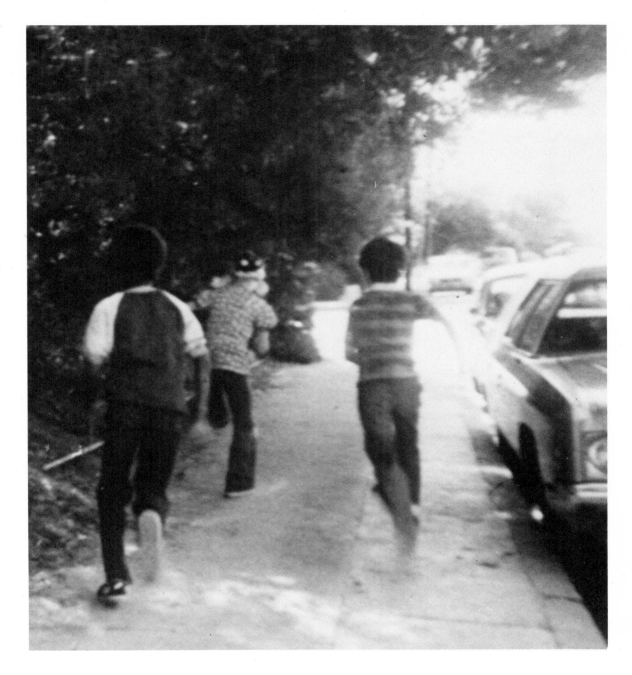

off after her. It turned into more of a race than a chase as
they neared Petey's house.

     Petey cut across the lawn and called, "Bye, guys."

     "See you later, Pete."

     "Ga-byeee," Kelly chirped.

Petey ran into the kitchen, the door slamming behind him. "Anybody home?" he called.

"We're up in your room, honey," his mom answered. "Your lunch is on the counter."

Petey gulped down the glass of milk and wiped his mouth on his sleeve. He grabbed the sandwich off the plate, then stopped to check the cookie jar. It was chock full, much to his delight. His mom must have spent the morning baking. She hadn't done that in a long time. Either it was too hot, or she was too tired. He bit into one of the cookies. It was still warm and chewy, and had raisins and nuts and little bumps in it. Mmmm. He ate another one, took two more for the road, and ran up the stairs.

A big carton was propped against the wall in the hall-way. Petey read the printing on the carton.

THIS SIDE UP

**Youth-Craft
Fine Makers Of Juvenile Furniture
Pine Crib**

He gave the crib a dirty look. When he reached his bedroom, he stood in the doorway and looked around. All of his furniture was in the middle of the room, covered with big cloths. Three of the walls were yellow now. The wall where his bed had been was still blue and had a big splotch of plaster in the middle of it.

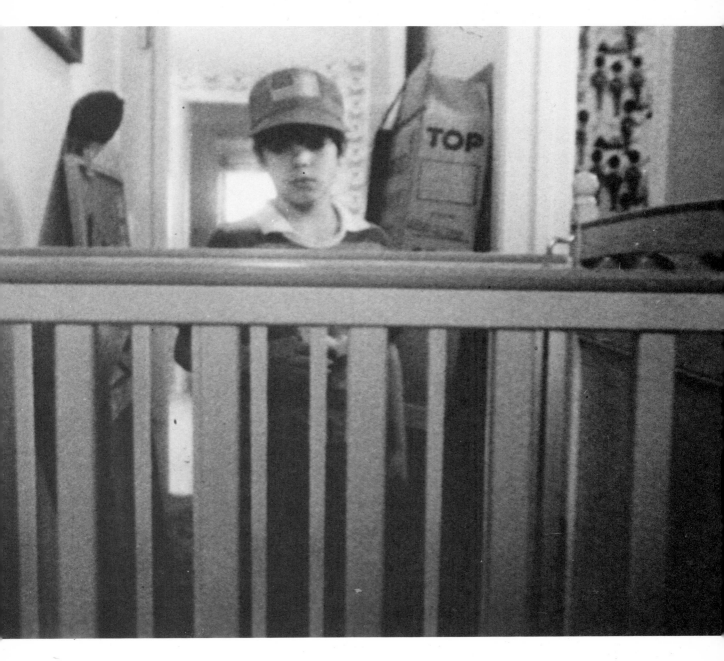

His mom was sitting on his bed. She looked hot
and wilted. She smiled at Petey. Gesturing around the room,
she said, "Well, how do you like it so far?"

Petey didn't like it. He bit into his sandwich and shrugged.

"Well," Mrs. Evans said, "It'll look better when it's all done. Come and sit next to me." He went over and sat down, and she put her arm around his shoulder.

Mr. Evans was prying open a can of paint. "How was the game?"

"We won," Petey said flatly. He didn't feel like talking about it. He finished his sandwich and bit into one of the cookies. "These cookies are fantastic, Mom."

Mr. Evans leaned against the dresser and winked at his wife. She winked back, then turned to Petey.

"Fantastic, huh?" she said. "I wasn't sure you'd like them when you found out what was in them."

Petey looked puzzled and examined the cookie more closely. "Why?" he said. "All those raisins and nuts. . . ."

"And Whammo Flakes," Mrs. Evans said.

"Huh?"

"You do remember the Whammo Flakes, don't you, honey?" She was obviously enjoying herself. She leaned against the headboard and giggled. Petey hadn't heard her giggle in a long time. It made him laugh. She reached over and gave him a big bear hug.

Mr. Evans chuckled at them. He walked over to the blue wall and ran his fingers over the plastered spot. "I think it's dry enough to paint over now."

Petey stood up. "Hey, that's where my hat hook was."

"I know," his dad said. "It left quite a hole in the wall."

"Aren't you going to put my hook back up?" Petey asked.

"No. The crib is going on this wall."

"But, Dad, you promised I could put everything back where it was."

"Pete, we can put the hook on another wall."

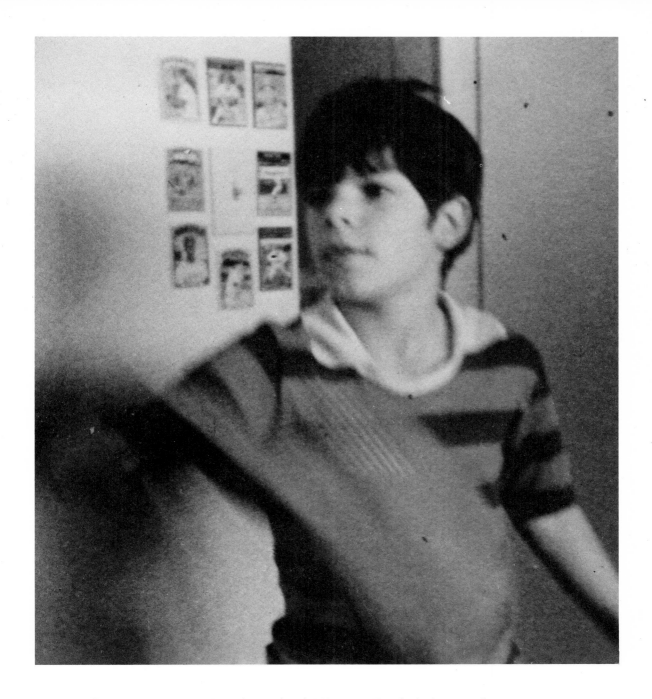

Petey was getting frantic. "Please, Dad, it has to be on that wall or it won't be in line with the light switch. See? When I come in, I hit the light and hook the hat." He demonstrated, flinging his hat, which hit the white spot like a bulls-eye.

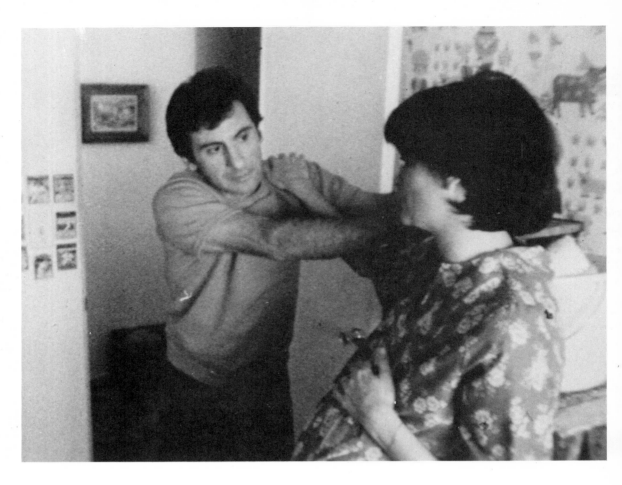

"Ohh, Jim," Mrs. Evans said.

Mr. Evans picked up the hat and put it on Petey's head. "Look, sport," he said, "that's really the best wall for the crib."

"The crib," Petey yelled. "The crib!! That's all that's important. That dumb crib!"

"Ohh, Petey," Mrs. Evans said. She looked as though she were going to cry.

Petey ran out of the room, tears streaming down his face. His dad called after him, but he kept running, down the stairs, through the house, and out into the yard.

Up in his room, Mr. and Mrs. Evans were bewildered.

"I think Pete's really fed up, Anne."

She nodded. "The hook goes back where it was, Jim. We'll put the crib on another wall."

Petey ran down the street, angry and frustrated. As he turned the corner, he spotted Oscar and Kelly. They ran to meet him.

"Hey, you said you weren't gonna play this afternoon," Kelly yelled.

"I changed my mind," Petey mumbled. He hoped they wouldn't notice he'd been crying.

Oscar was eating a popsicle that was melting fast in the heat and dripping down the front of his shirt. He slurped. "What's the matter with you?"

Petey didn't answer.

"Did you get the baby's room ready?" Kelly asked.

"My mom and dad are doing it," Petey said. "Could we talk about something else?"

Oscar stopped slurping. "Boy, you're really touchy."

"I'm just sick of babies right now, okay?"

"I know what," Kelly said. "When the stork comes, why don't you give him the wrong directions." She cupped her hands around her mouth and shouted, "The Evanses live four blocks down that-away!" She pointed in the direction opposite Petey's house.

Oscar slurped. "You probably think that's where babies do come from."

"Well," Kelly said, "my sister said they found me at the dump, but I don't believe her."

"I do," Petey said.

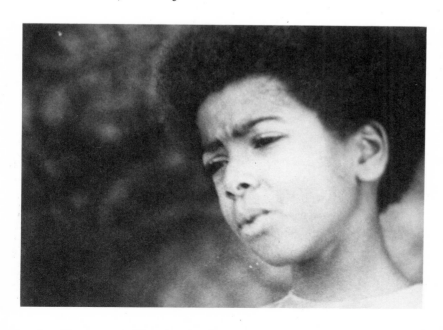

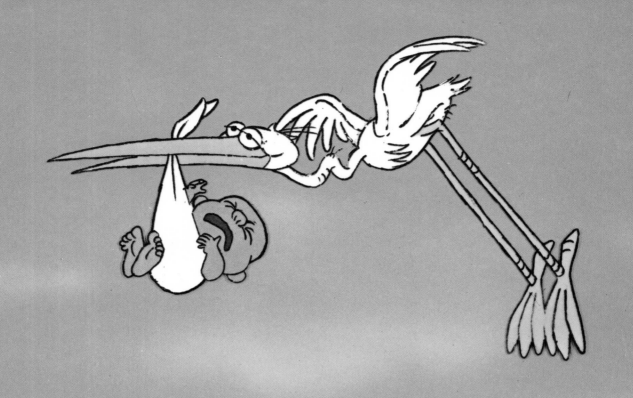

"Thanks a lot." Kelly jabbed Petey's shoulder.

"Okay, smarty." Oscar said to Kelly. "Where *do* babies come from ?"

"If you don't know, I'm certainly not going to tell you," she answered.

Oscar frowned. He wished Kelly had given him a

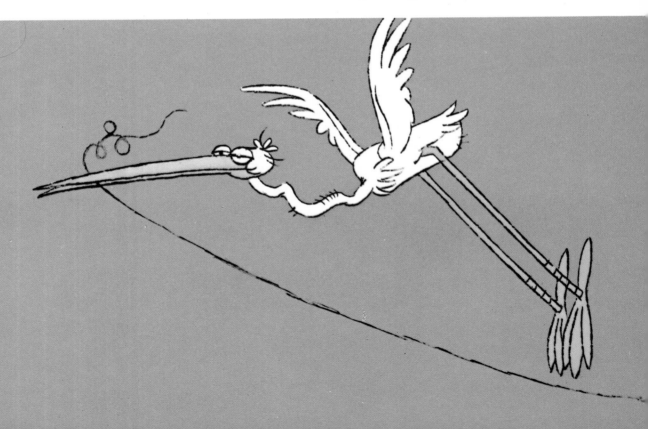

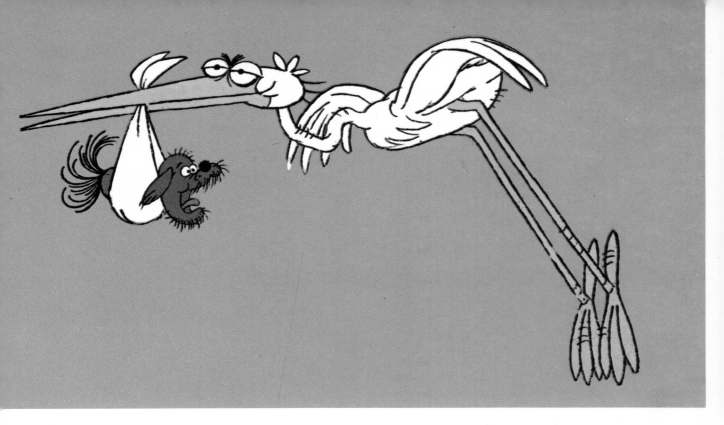

straight answer. This business about the stork puzzled him.
He imagined a stork soaring through the sky,
carrying a baby in his beak. Another stork flew by, carrying
a baby elephant, then another with a baby skunk,
and another with a puppy.

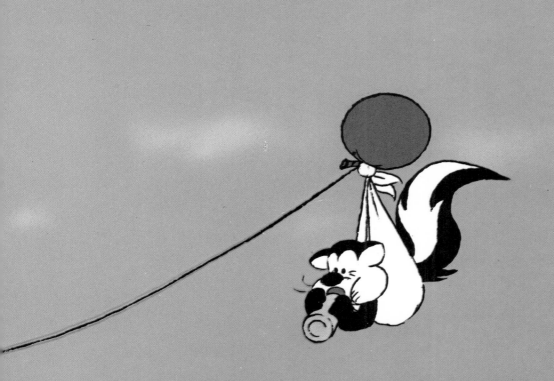

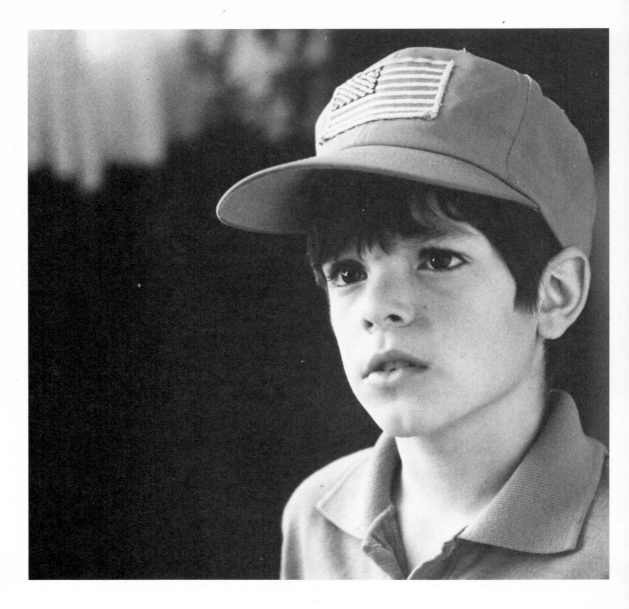

Good grief, Oscar! What a wonderful
imagination you have. Come on, now.
The stork doesn't really bring babies . . .
or elephants, or skunks, or puppies.

Oscar shook his head, coming out of his daydream, and
concentrated on his popsicle.

  Petey tugged at the brim of his hat, pulling it
down over his forehead. "Well, I know one thing," he said.
"My mom's going to the hospital to get her baby."

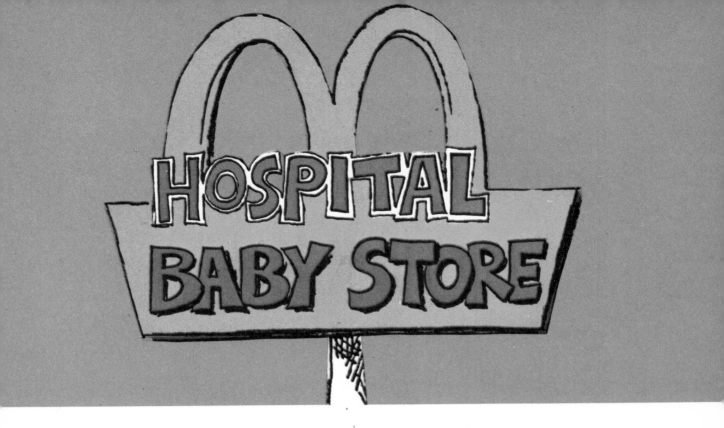

Petey thought about the hospital. He'd never been inside one. In his imagination it looked like a drive-in restaurant. There were golden arches and a neon sign that said HOSPITAL BABY STORE. Under that, another sign said, OVER ONE BILLION SOLD.

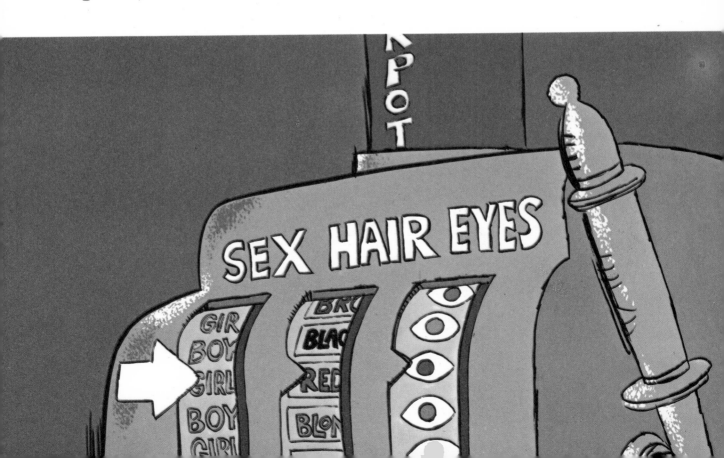

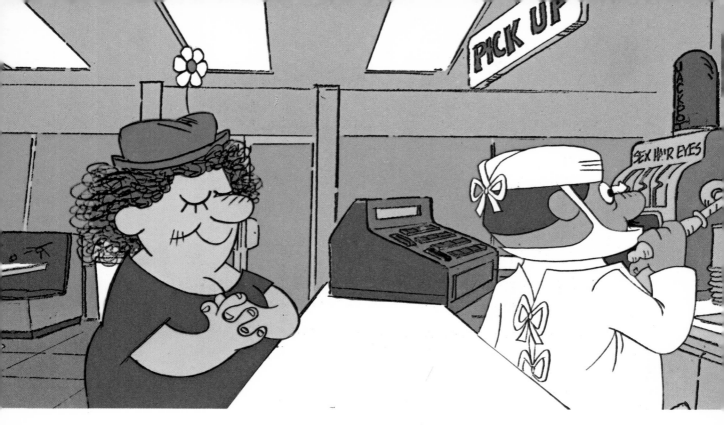

A lady opened the door and walked up to a long
counter.

The man behind the counter said, "May I help you,
m'am?"

The lady smiled and said, "Yes, please. I'd like a baby
girl, a chocolate shake, and a side order of fries."

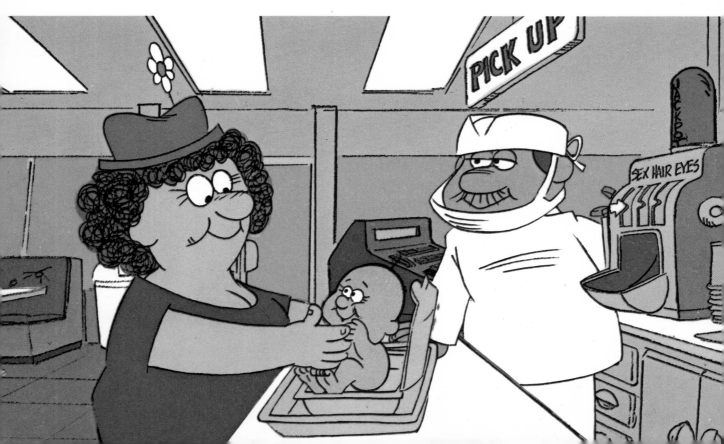

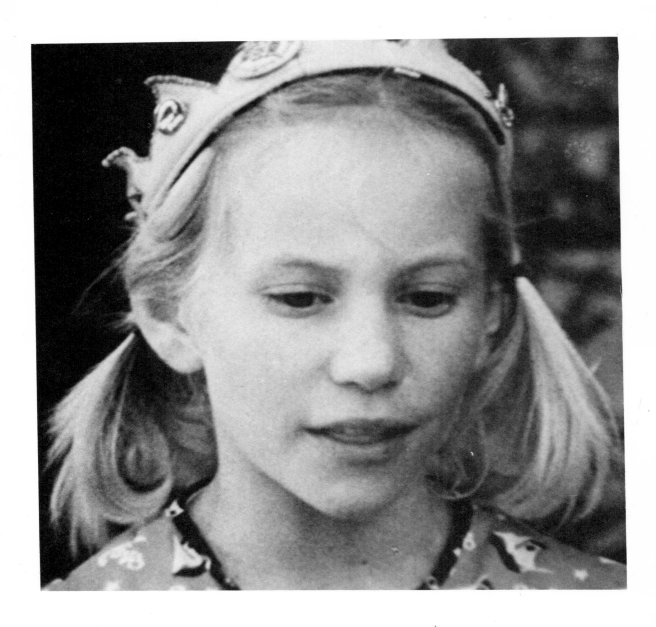

Gracious, Petey, you are definitely confused.

Kelly had been doing cartwheels, but was listening carefully to what Petey and Oscar were saying. She flipped over one more time, then stood with her hands on her hips. "Well, of course you get babies at the hospital," she said. "But the baby comes out of the mother's stomach."

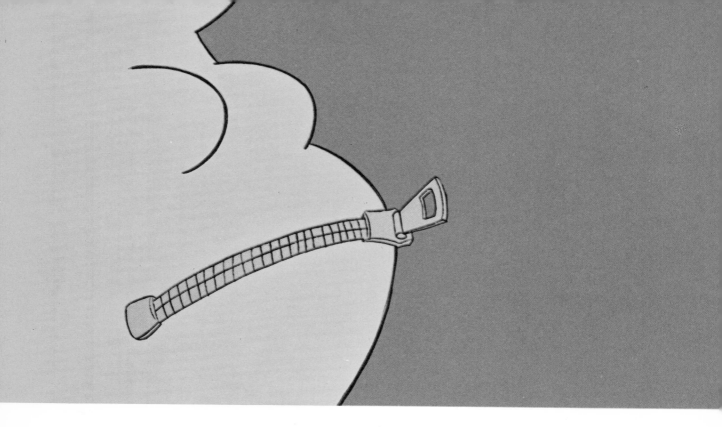

She'd heard that piece of information somewhere, but never bothered to find out the rest of the story. So she made up the ending. She imagined a stomach with a zipper in it. The zipper opened, and a baby poked it's head out, smiled, and said, "Goo," then stuck it's thumb in it's mouth.

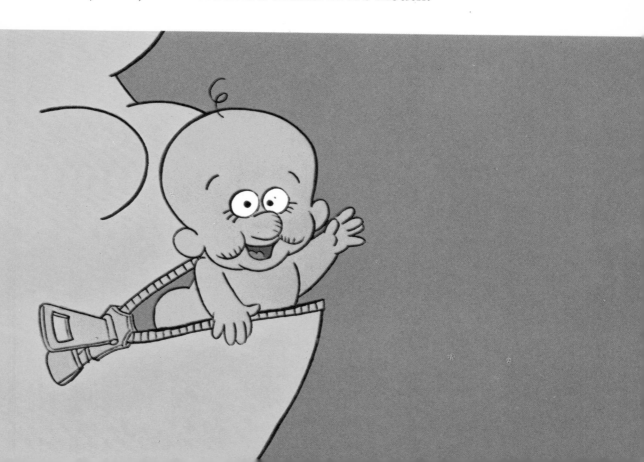

*Okay, Kel, you're getting warm, but your
facts are still a little mixed up.*

"Well," Petey said, "there's gotta be more to it."

"Lots more," Oscar said, slurping.

Kelly studied both boys, then sighed. "All right, gentlemen," she announced. "I'll tell you all about the birds and the bees . . . but not until you get a little older."

She laughed and ran away from them. Petey took off after her, but Oscar stopped walking.

Part of his popsicle had fallen on his sneaker. He studied it for a second, then flicked his toe. The little glob of ice landed in the bushes. Meanwhile, the other half of the popsicle was running down his arm, leaving sticky purple streaks. The whole thing was beginning to fascinate him. He probably would have stood there all afternoon, but Kelly noticed Oscar had stopped moving.

"For crying out loud, Oscar," she yelled. "Can't you even eat a popsicle right? Come on, Petey. I don't even want to be seen with him."

Petey laughed. Oscar really looked funny. He ran back to him and put his arm around Oscar's shoulder. They caught up with Kelly, and Petey said, "Kel, I'd like you to meet my friend, Oscar the grape."

On Monday morning, Petey sat in the waiting room in Doctor Smith's office and watched the rain pelt down outside the window.

"Well, there goes the ole ball game," he said.

Mrs. Evans handed him a magazine. "According to the weatherman," she said, "the rain might last for a couple of days. Dad hopes it will, because the lawn is really drying up."

Petey moaned and tossed the magazine aside. He didn't care if the lawn died of thirst. If it rained, he wouldn't be able to play ball.

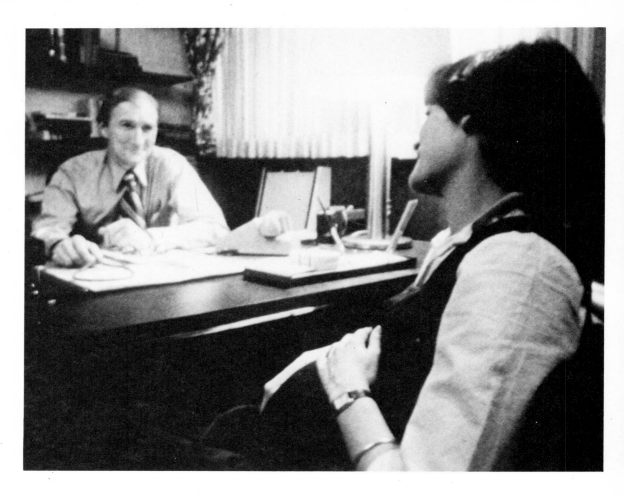

"Peter Evans."

Dr. Smith's nurse motioned to him. He and Mrs. Evans stood up and walked toward the examining rooms. In the hallway, they bumped into the doctor.

"Hi, Pete," Dr. Smith said. "Go on in, and strip down to your underwear. I'll be right in." He turned to Mrs. Evans and took her arm. "Come and sit down, Anne," he said, and led her into his office. He helped her into a chair, then sat at his desk, facing her.

"Now how are you feeling?" he asked.

"Anxious . . . and fat," she said. "Lendon, I'm kind of worried about Petey. He's been a little mopey lately. I'm pretty sure it's because of the baby. . . . " She paused.

"Well, Anne," Dr. Smith said, "new babies can really upset a household, even before they arrive."

"I know," she said, "and so can their mothers. I've been an absolute bear lately, both to Petey and to Jim."

"Well, hang in there " Dr. Smith said. "It'll soon be over, then the real fun begins!" He smiled at her, then grew serious. "Have you discussed childbirth with Petey at all?"

"Well, sort of. . . ." Mrs. Evans answered.

"You know, part of his moodiness could be caused by the fact that he doesn't understand what's happening," Dr. Smith explained. "Don't you think now is a good time to tell him?"

"Isn't he a little young?" Mrs. Evans asked. "It's not the easiest thing to explain to a child."

"I don't think he's too young," the doctor said. "He should know more than just 'Mommy's going to the hospital.' If you like, I have a good film about reproduction. I could show and tell."

"I'd like that," Mrs. Evans said.

Dr. Smith stood up. "Fine," he said. "You wait here, and Petey and I will set something up." He patted her hand and went out of the room.

Petey stood on the scale in the examining room. He hoped the scale would say he weighed a hundred pounds. He was wearing only his undershorts, and every so often he shivered. Fortunately, he had on his red cap, so at least his head was warm. He wondered if all the goose pimples on his arms made him weigh more.

Dr. Smith came into the room. He adjusted the weights on the scale. "Hmmm," he said. "You've gained seven pounds since last year, and you're two inches taller. Now, hop up on the table."

"When will I weigh a hundred pounds?" Petey asked.

Dr. Smith smiled. "Not for a few years yet. Probably when your new baby is about three years old. By the way, what do you want, a brother or a sister?"

Petey shrugged. "It doesn't matter what I want."

"Oh, Petey," Dr. Smith said warmly. "It sounds as though you might be having a kind of rough time at home. I bet your mom has been a little grouchy lately."

Petey nodded.

"Is she tired a lot, too?" Dr. Smith asked.

"Yeah." Petey said. "She's always taking a nap."

"Listen, Petey. Your mom's been carrying that baby around for nine months. She's pooped!"

Petey whistled. "Nine months?"

"Uh-huh," Dr. Smith said. "And it's the end of the summer, so the heat makes her uncomfortable, too. She's just as eager to have the baby born as you are."

"I'm not eager," Petey said. "We don't need a baby."

"Petey, I've known you for a long time. In fact, I can remember the day you were born. You made your mom and dad so happy. Now the new baby will make you all happy. It's fun to have a brother or sister."

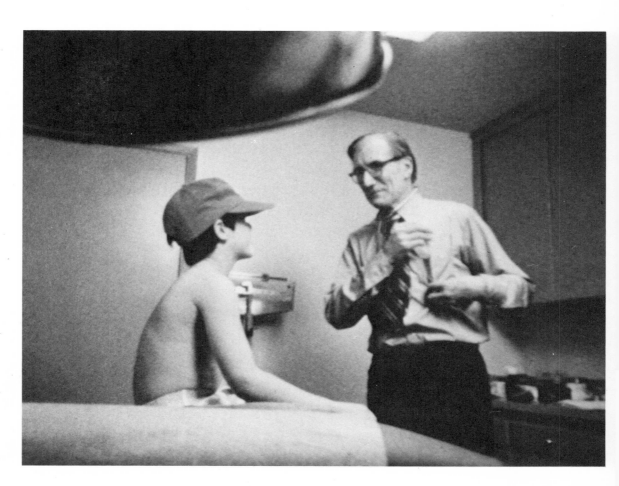

"All they can do is cry and wet their pants," Petey said. "What's fun about that?"

Dr. Smith laughed. "That was all you could do for a while, too. But now, you're going to be a big brother, and that's an important job. You can help teach the baby to talk, and walk and . . . even play baseball."

"What if he's a girl?" Petey asked.

"Then you can teach her to play baseball, and she can go around bragging about it. She'll say 'My big brother weighs over a hundred pounds and he taught me to play baseball.'"

Petey laughed.

After the doctor finished the examination, he told Petey to get dressed. "Your mom's waiting in my office," he said. "We talked for a while, and I told her I've got a movie about babies and how they're born. It's like a cartoon. Would you like to see it?"

"Sure!" Petey said.

"Great," Dr. Smith said. "We'll ask your mom if you can come down Wednesday afternoon, when the office is closed. How's that?"

"It's okay with me," Petey said. "Can I bring my friends Oscar and Kelly?"

"Sure," Dr. Smith said. "As long as it's okay with their parents. I love an audience! Come on, let's go tell your mom."

Wednesday afternoon Petey, Oscar, and Kelly met before going over to the medical building. They sat on a curb for a while.

Kelly was trying hard not to show her excitement. She looked up at the gloomy sky and sighed. "If it were a nicer day, I'd be playing ball, you know. I wouldn't be coming here."

Petey rolled his eyes. "Come on, Kel. You would too."

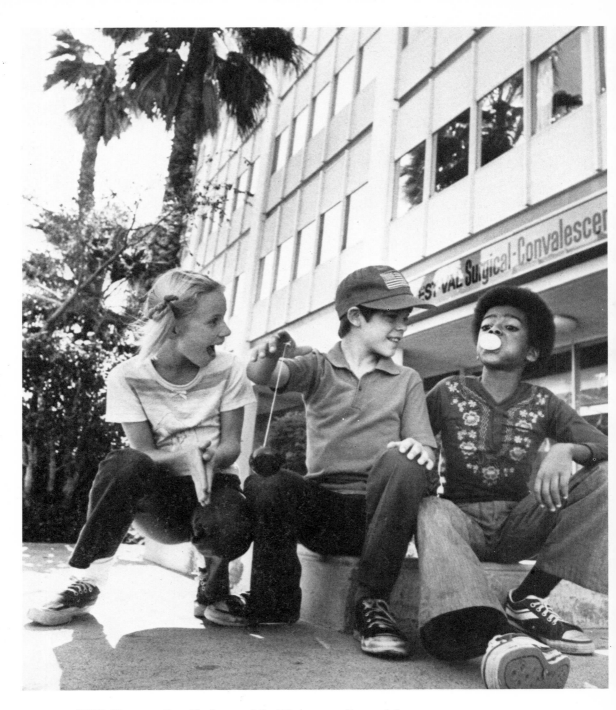

"Well, maybe," she said. "I guess I could brush up on my facts a little. What did your mom say about this, Oscar?"

"My mom's working," Oscar said, "but Dad told Dr. Smith maybe he'd come, too."

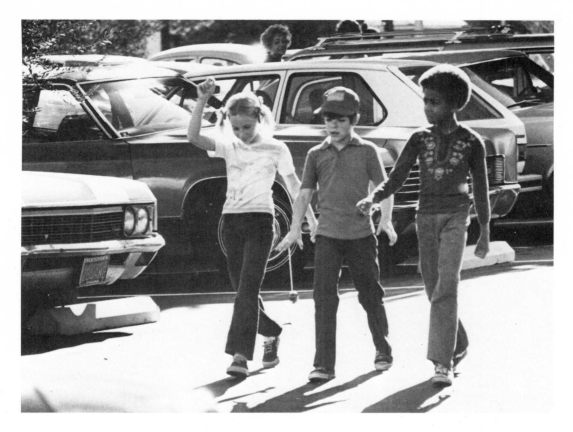

They laughed, then they got up, walked
through the parking lot, and ran up the sidewalk in front
of the building.

Kelly held the front door open with a grand,
sweeping bow, which both boys ignored. They raced past her
and skidded to a halt in front of the elevator. Oscar
leaned against the 'door open' button and blew a bubble.

"Quit leaning on the button, dummy," Kelly yelled.
"You'll break the doors."

Just as she spoke, the doors opened and the children
scrambled inside the elevator. They watched the number
lights change as they passed each floor. Then, with a ping,
they stopped, and the doors opened.

Petey and Kelly bolted out, but Oscar sauntered out,
taking his time. He grabbed the elevator door before it
closed, and pushed the wall button. The door sprung open.
He did this three or four times, then a loud buzz
sounded, and he jumped.

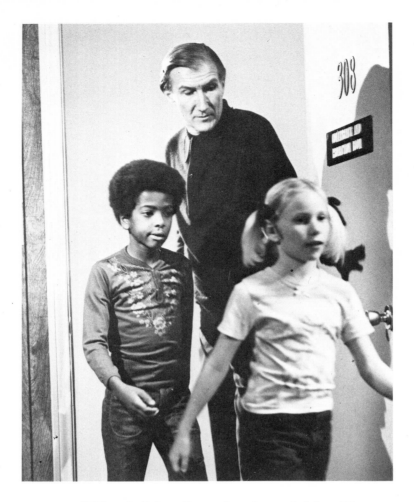

"Uh-oh," he thought sheepishly. He turned and
ran down the hall to where Petey and Kelly were standing
with Dr. Smith.

"Hi, Oscar," Dr. Smith said. "I'm glad you all could
come. Are you ready for the show?"

"Yeah!" they cried. "Let's go!"

Dr. Smith took a bunch of keys out of his
pocket and unlocked a door marked MEDICAL CENTER
SCREENING ROOM.

The children were surprised when they stepped
inside. The room was very large. In the center, was
a long table flanked by two rows of chairs. At the far end of the
room was a huge motion-picture screen.

"Wow!" Oscar said. "Look at the size of that screen!"

Even Kelly was impressed. For once, she was speechless.

"Is this going to be like a real movie?" Petey asked.

"Absolutely," said Dr. Smith. "Now pull up some chairs, nice and close, and we'll get started."

"Ooo-kay!" they squealed, and scrambled for seats.

Dr. Smith stood in front of the screen, facing them. "Lady and gentlemen, welcome to Anatomy Street!" he announced.

The children clapped and cheered.

Dr. Smith bowed. "Thank you all very much. As you know, the film we're going to see is about how babies are born. I'll explain it as we go along, and please feel free to ask questions if there's anything you don't understand."

He sat down next to a small mechanical box with a lot of buttons on it. He pressed a button and the room went dark.

Then the screen lit up.

"You are about to see the most extraordinary of all creations," Dr. Smith said.

Just then, a silhouette of a woman appeared on the screen.

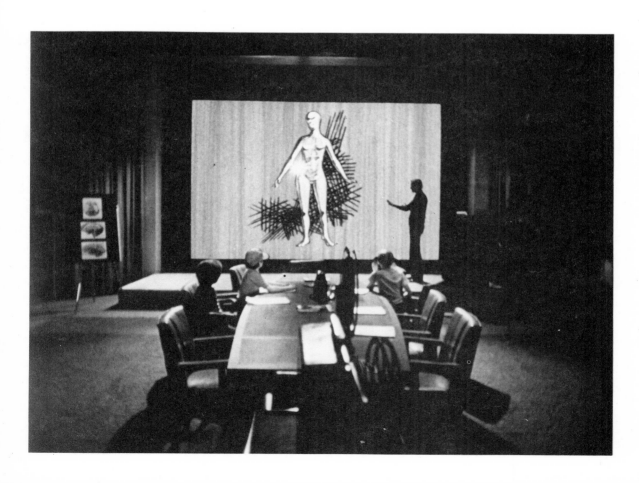

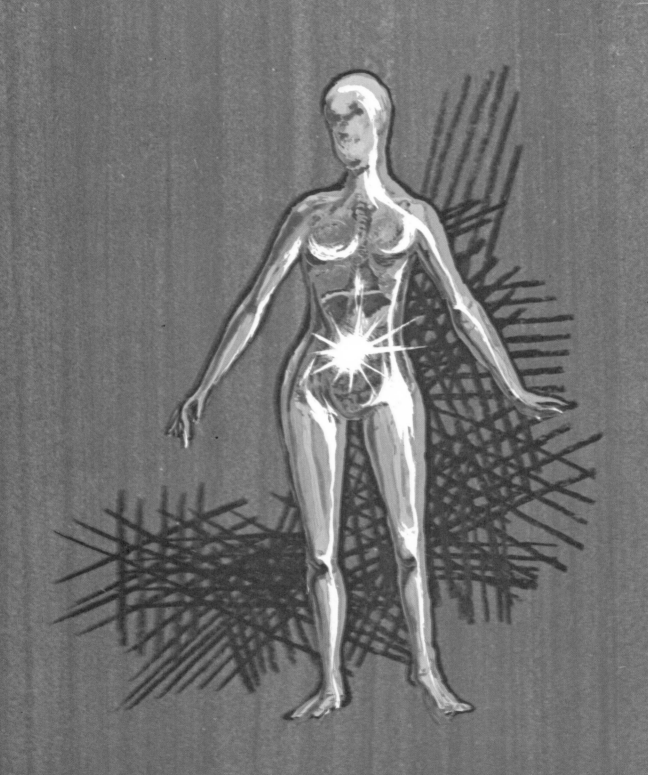

" . . . the human female body," Dr. Smith continued.

"That's it?" said Kelly.

"What's so great about a woman?" Oscar asked.

"Well," Dr. Smith said, "for one thing, only a woman can give birth to another human being. Now let's get on with the show!"

With a flourish of music and explosion of color, the silhouette changed to a figure revealing the inside of a woman's body—like an X-ray picture. The figure grew larger and filled the screen. Then, just the area where the reproductive organs are was visible.

"Hey, what's all that?" asked Petey.

"What you see is the female reproductive system," Dr. Smith explained.

"Huh?"

"Okay, okay," continued the doctor. "Simply speaking, these are the parts in a woman's body that work together to make a baby."

Movement on the screen showed the *fimbriae* gently swaying.

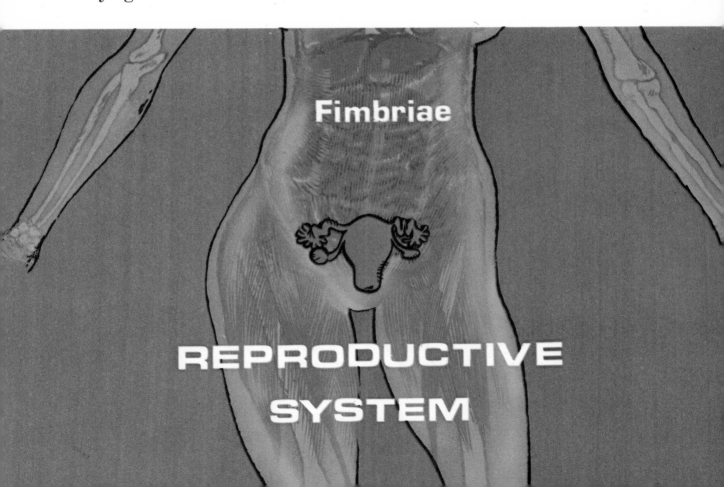

Fimbriae

REPRODUCTIVE SYSTEM

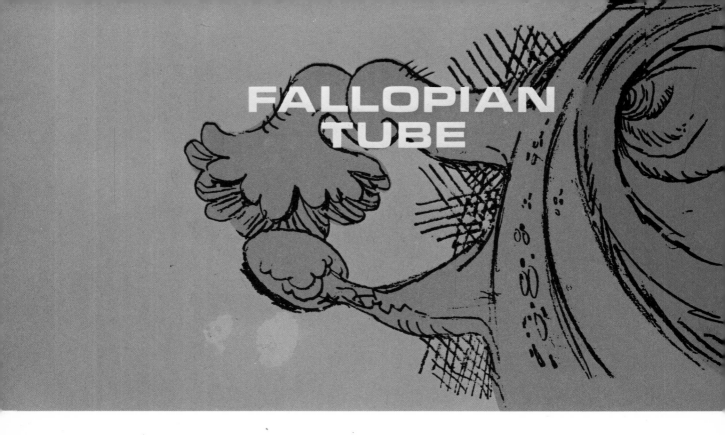

FALLOPIAN TUBE

Dr. Smith continued to speak. "At the end of the tube on the left are the *fimbriae*. The tube is called the *fallopian tube*. Just below the fimbriae, that kind of lumpy, oval-shaped thing is called the *ovary*. The ovary holds eggs, and each month it releases an egg. Watch closely."

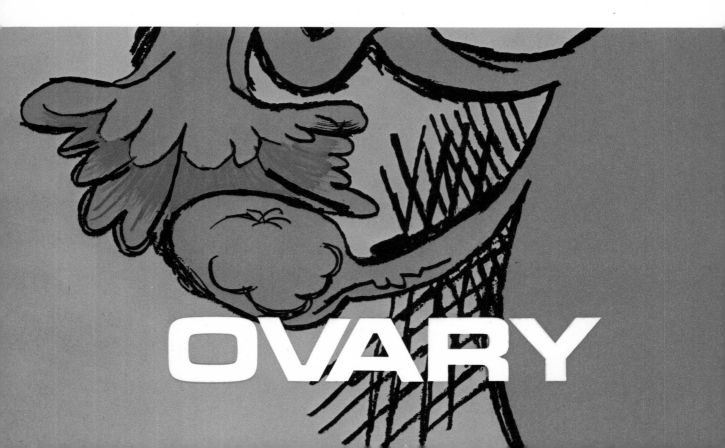

OVARY

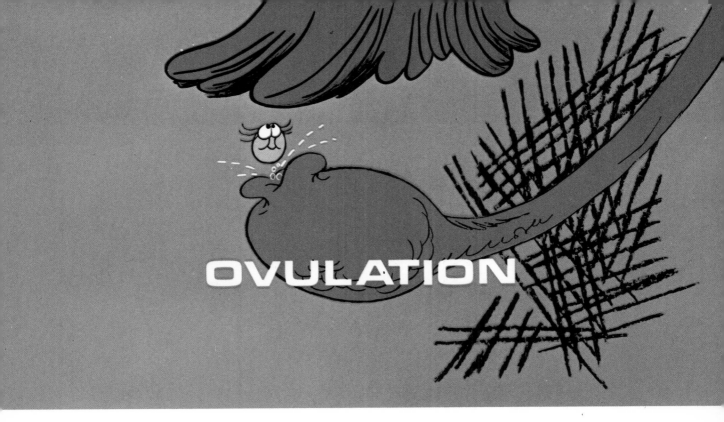

OVULATION

The ovary looked like a bulging sack of potatoes. The little bulges were moving, and suddenly a tiny egg fell out with a little pop. The egg was quickly swept up by the fimbriae, into the fallopian tube.

Dr. Smith explained, "You'll notice another fallopian tube and ovary on the right side. Each month, one of the ovaries releases an egg. They take turns. One month the left side, the next month the right side. This process is called *ovulation*."

"Is the egg like a regular egg—like chickens lay?" Petey asked.

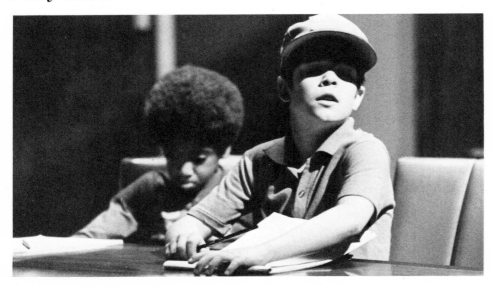

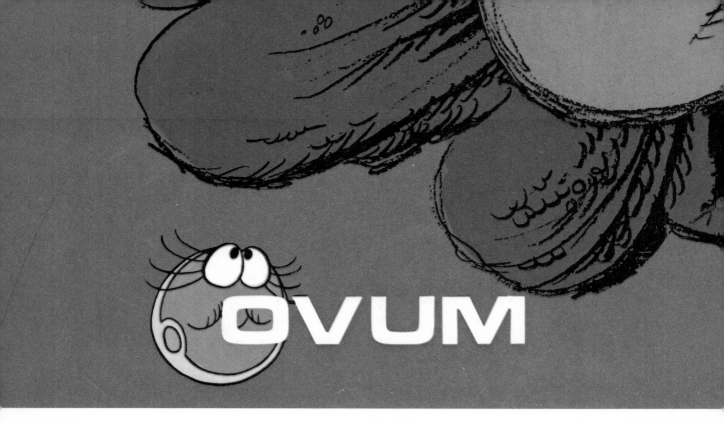

OVUM

"Not really," said Dr. Smith. "Technically, the egg is called the *ovum*, and it's so tiny, you would barely be able to see it."

"Is the egg the baby?" asked Oscar.

"Yes and no," said Dr. Smith. "The egg is the mother's contribution to the beginning of life."

"What's the father's?" asked Petey.

Before Dr. Smith could answer, some new activity developed on the screen.

"Hey," said Oscar, "look at all the tadpoles!"

Hundreds of squiggly little "tadpoles" swam across the screen.

"There's the father's contribution, right there," Dr. Smith said. "but they aren't tadpoles. They're called *sperm*."

Oscar was amazed. "You mean *all* those sperm and just *one* little egg make the baby?"

Dr. Smith laughed. "No," he said. "Just one sperm joining the egg will make the baby."

"Which sperm?" Petey asked.

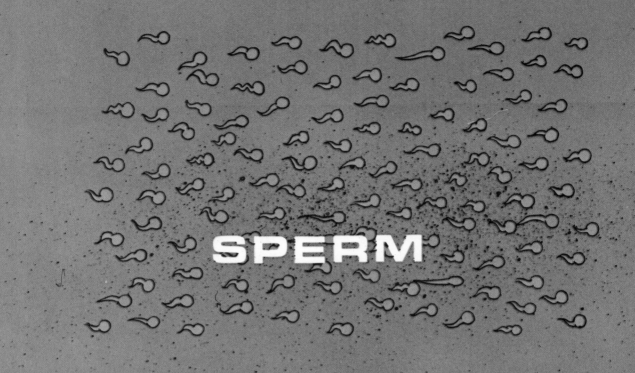

SPERM

"I bet I know," Kelly said. "The first one to get to the egg is the winner. Right?"

"Right!" said Dr. Smith.

Petey was puzzled. "How did the sperm get from the father to the mother?" he asked.

Dr. Smith paused. "Good question, Pete. . . . Well, this happens when a man and a woman are making love. It's also called having intercourse. The man and the woman come so close together that a part of his body, called the penis, fits into a part of her body, called the vagina. It's during this loving moment that the penis releases the sperm into the woman's body."

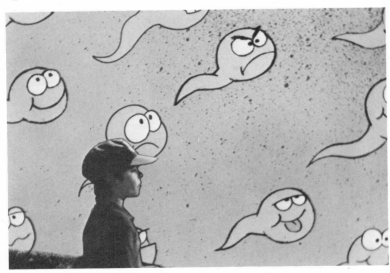

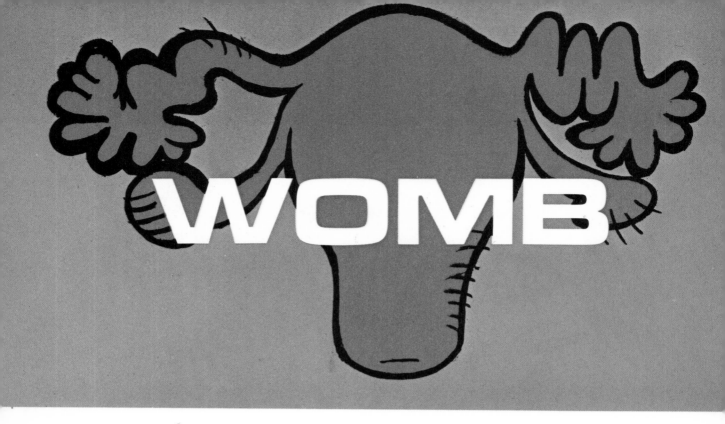

On the screen, the sperm continued to swim up through the vagina and cervix, into the uterus.

Dr. Smith continued to explain as they watched. "Some of the sperm are slowing down. They've entered what's called the *uterus*, or *womb*, and are heading toward the fallopian tube. Watch that one

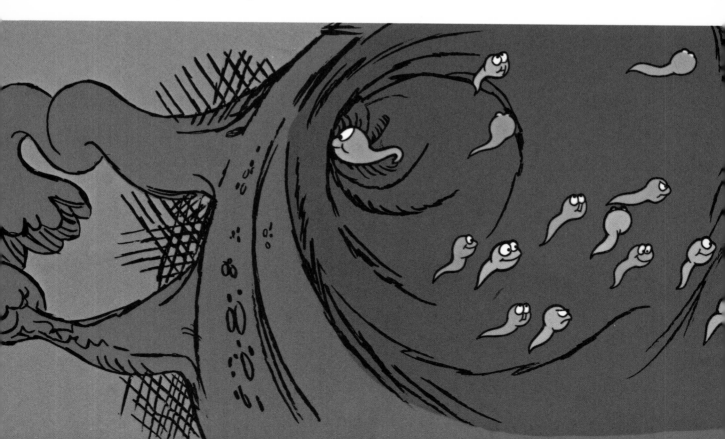

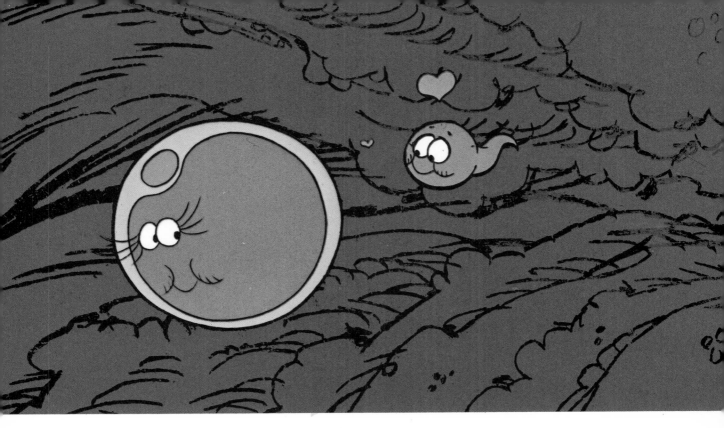

near the top of the uterus. It's heading right for the egg."

 The egg, traveling from one direction, was quickly moving toward the sperm coming from the other direction. They were almost ready to meet when Oscar yelled, "Look out! They're going to crash!"

 "Let's hope they do," Dr. Smith said.

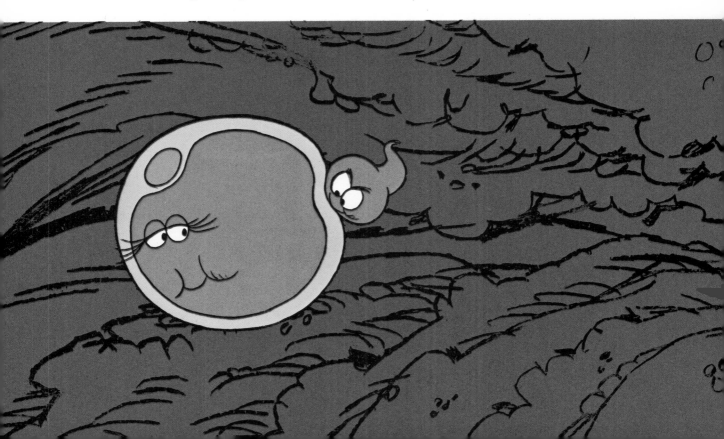

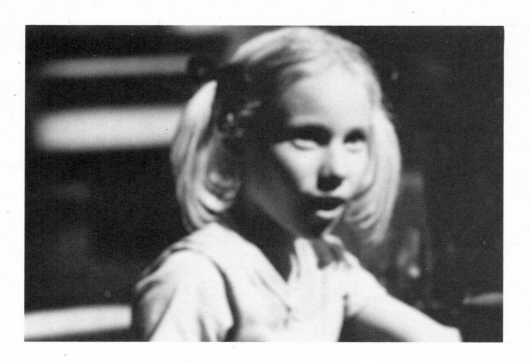

"Why?" the children chimed.

"Because this is the first step in the creation of life," the doctor said.

The music got louder, and suddenly the sperm and the egg collided.

"Well, they crashed," Kelly said.

"They sure did," said Dr. Smith. "That crash has a special name. It's called *fertilization*."

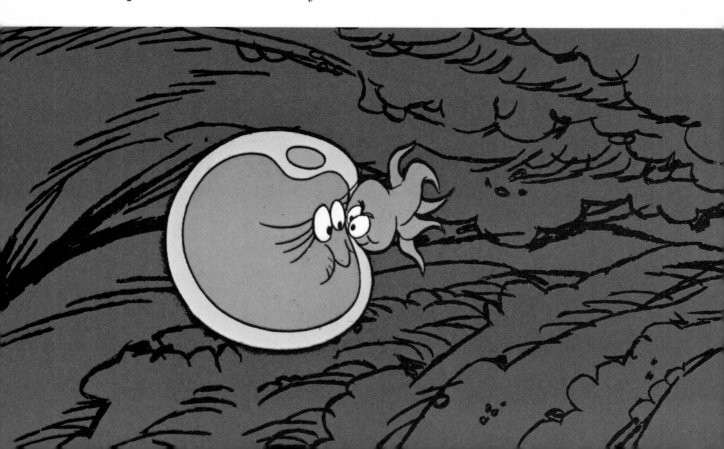

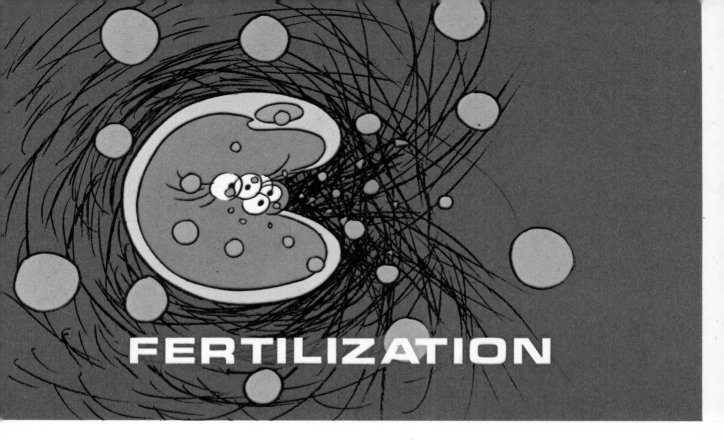

FERTILIZATION

As soon as the sperm touched the egg, they united, then split into two still-connected cells.

"Oh, it broke," said Oscar.

The cell continued to divide into four, then eight sections, and on and on, until it looked like a bunch of grapes.

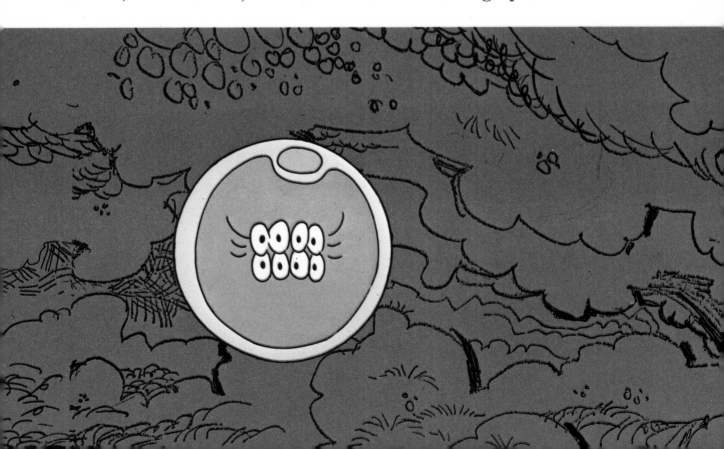

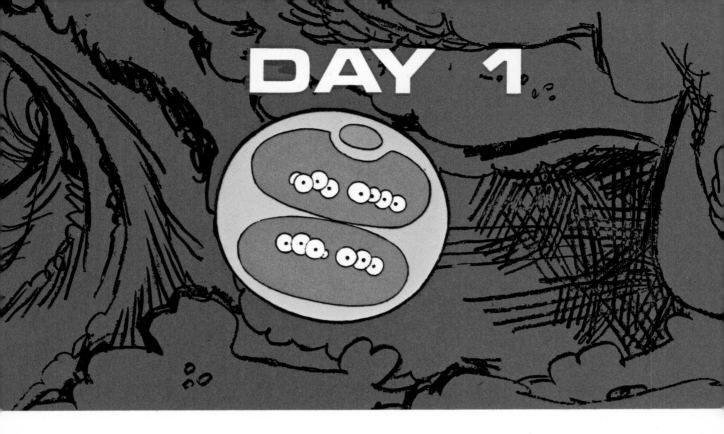

DAY 1

It moved gracefully out of the end of the fallopian
tube and down into the uterus.
   "My friends," said Dr. Smith, "you have
just witnessed the very beginning of a human life."
   The fertilized egg burrowed into the uterine lining.

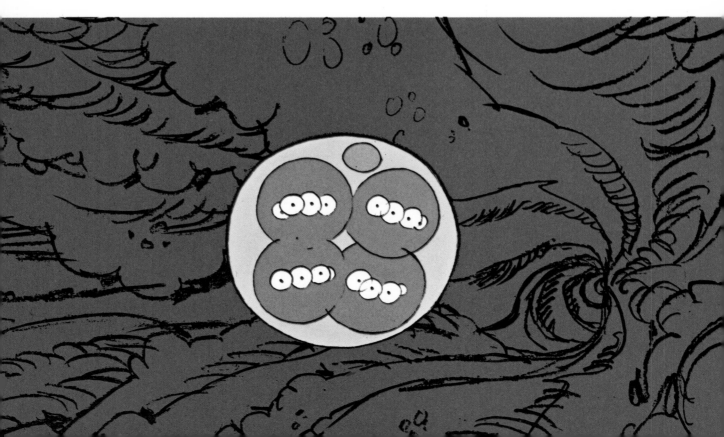

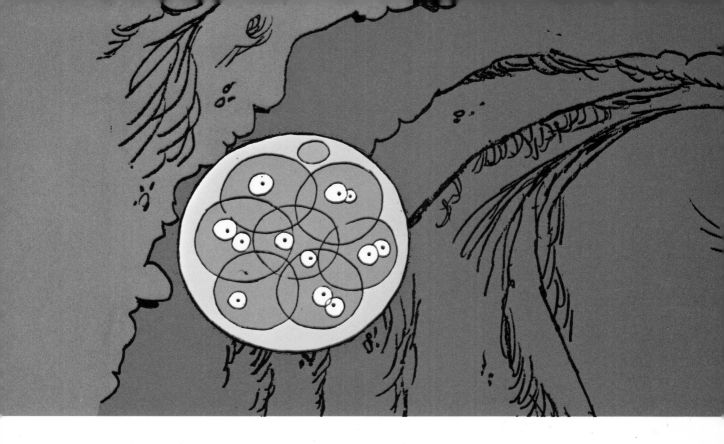

"Now it's stuck," said Petey.

"And that's where it will stay and grow until the baby is born," said the doctor.

"That bunch of blobs sure doesn't look like a brother or sister," Petey said, disappointed.

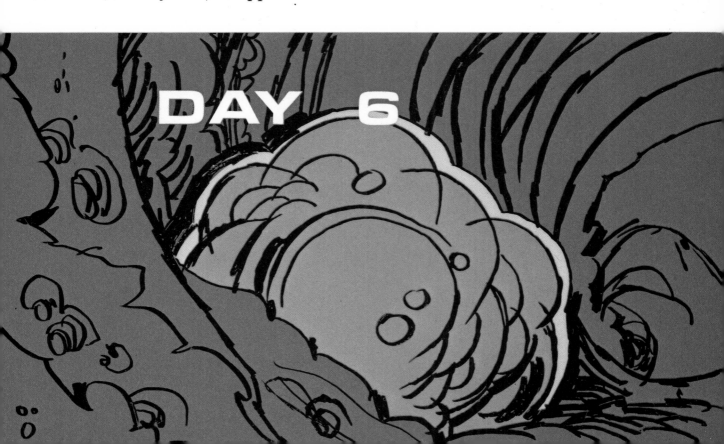

DAY 6

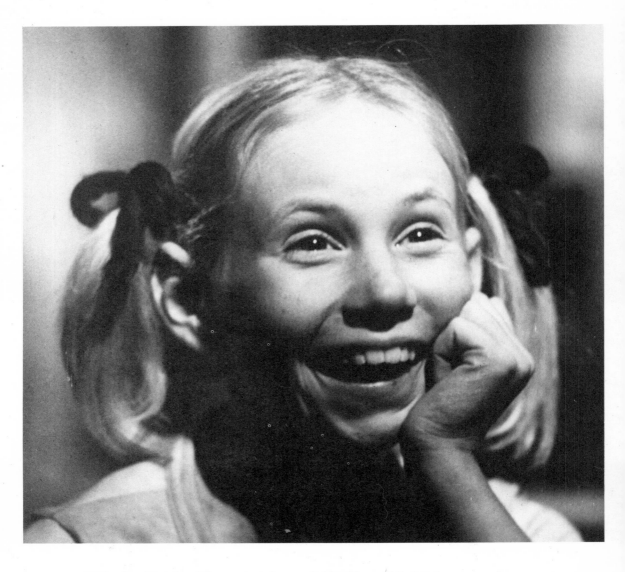

"Kind of looks like *my* sister." Kelly said dryly. Everybody laughed.

"Don't worry, Petey," said Dr. Smith. "It'll start to look like a baby. Let's speed things up, and I'll show you."

The doctor pressed a button. The film spun into a blur, then stopped. On the screen was a picture of the fetus at three months.

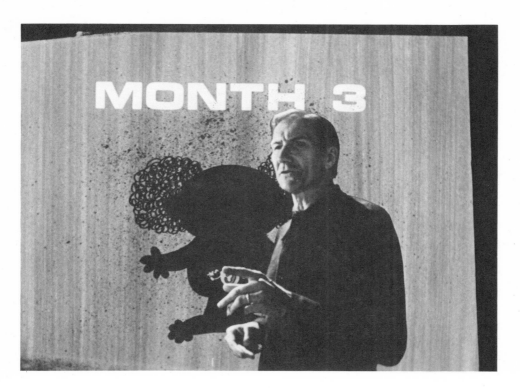

Dr. Smith spoke. "The baby has been growing inside his mother for three months, now. His little heart has started to beat, and you can already make out his face."

"Hey, he sort of looks like a baby," Petey said.

"It could be a she," Kelly said. "How big is *she* now, Dr. Smith?"

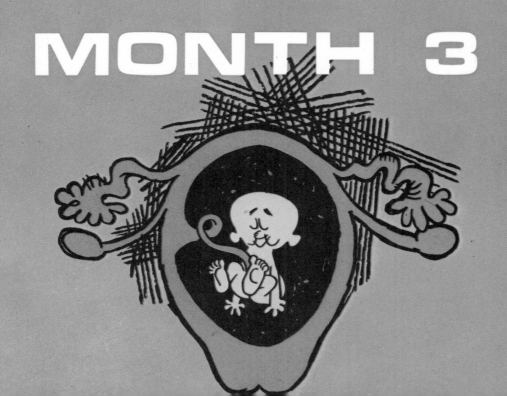

MONTH 6

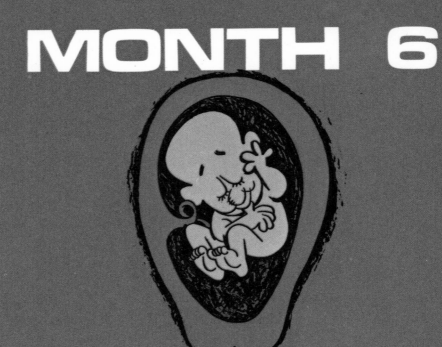

   "She . . . or he, is about the size of your fist,
Kelly," the doctor answered. "Notice that she, or he, already
has fingers and toes. Let's move ahead to when the
baby is six months old."
   He pressed a button again, and the film whirred
and stopped. The baby was larger and more active. It kicked
vigorously and did a somersault.
   The children were amazed.

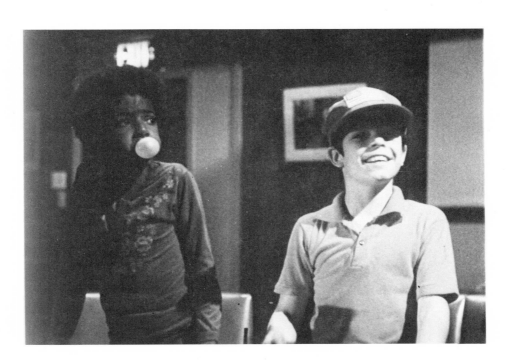

"Son of a gun," Oscar said. "Look at that!"

"My mom's baby's been kicking for a long time," Petey announced. "I've felt it."

"What did it feel like?" asked Kelly.

Petey was excited now. "Sort of like a big toe wiggling under the covers." They all laughed. "Honest, it really did. . . . I felt it!"

The baby settled down and seemed to be asleep with it's thumb in it's mouth.

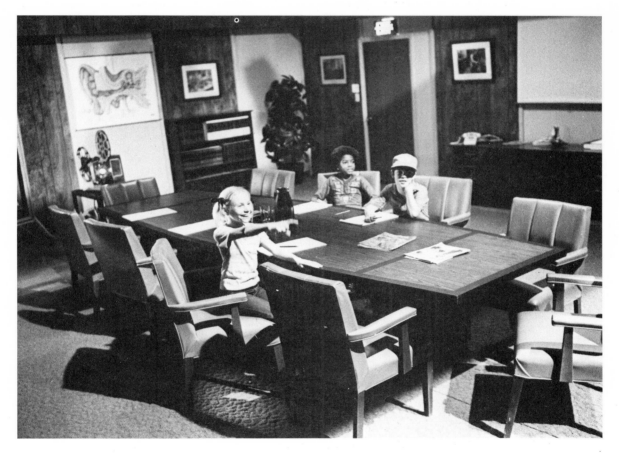

Kelly was beside herself. "Oh, I don't believe this . . . look at him . . . her. Hey, get your thumb out of your mouth. You'll ruin your teeth!"

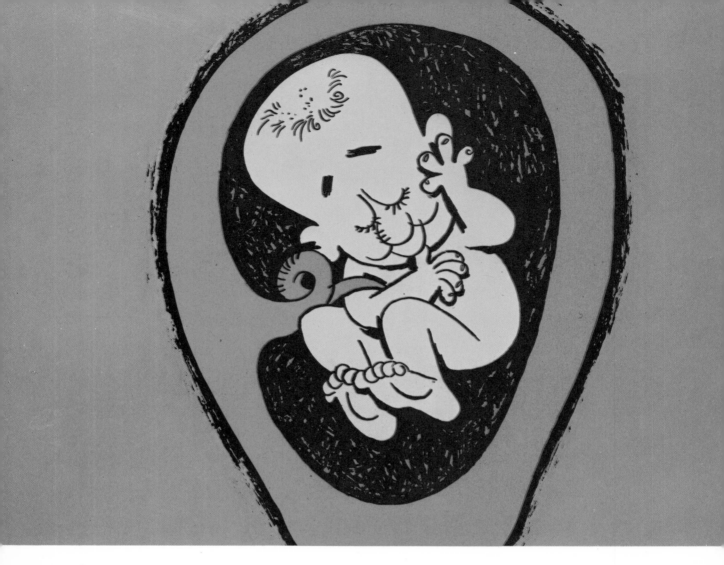

Dr. Smith chuckled. "No teeth, yet, Kelly,"
he said, "but the baby has almost everything else. Nails,
hair, the works."

Petey whispered. "Is he really sleeping?"

"Yes," said Dr. Smith. "They can get tired, too."

"Well," Kelly observed, "There's not much to do.
She's probably just bored."

"Is the baby ready to be born yet?" Oscar asked.

"Not yet," Dr. Smith answered. "He still has lots of
growing to do."

Petey was getting impatient. "Well, how much
longer?" he asked.

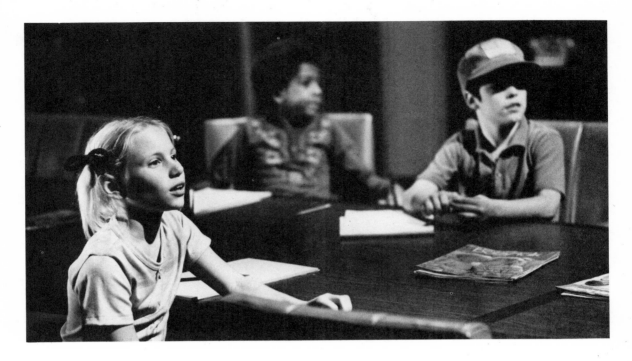

"You'll see," the doctor said. He pushed the button again, speeding up the film. "We'll see it at nine months, now."

The baby now was full grown. He was snugly packed into the womb, in an upside-down position, with his head pressed against the birth canal.

Kelly gasped. "Good grief, she's huge!!"

Oscar's eyes opened wide. "Son of a gun," he said. "Look at that! That kid must weigh five hundred pounds!"

"Nope," said Dr. Smith. "More like six or seven pounds, and he's only about as tall as your arm."

"How come he's standing on his head?" Petey said.

"He turned about a month ago, Petey," said the doctor. "That means he's getting ready to be born."

"You mean that's all there is to it?" said Oscar. "He just stands on his head and he's born?"

"Not quite," said Dr. Smith. "The walls of the uterus have very, very strong muscles in them. When it's

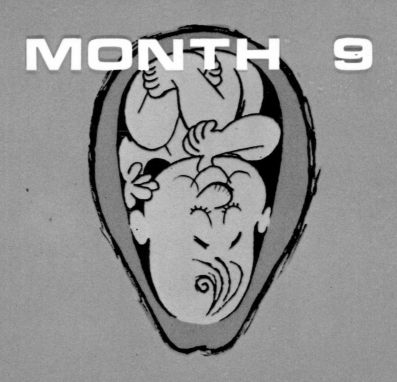

MONTH 9

time for the baby to be born, these muscles squeeze the baby down and out through the vagina and into the world."

Kelly made a strangulated, gagging noise, as though she were being squeezed too tightly. She grabbed her throat, coughed, and slid down into her chair.

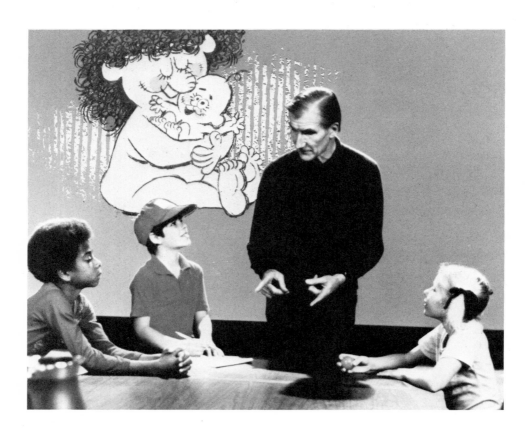

Oscar cuffed her in the arm.

"Quit showing off, Kel," said Petey.

"I was just pretending I was being born," said Kelly.

Dr. Smith laughed. "Well, I think you overdid it a little," he said. "Actually, it's not one long squeeze. It's more like a whole lot of pushes. They're called contractions."

Petey looked concerned. "Does that hurt the mother?" he asked.

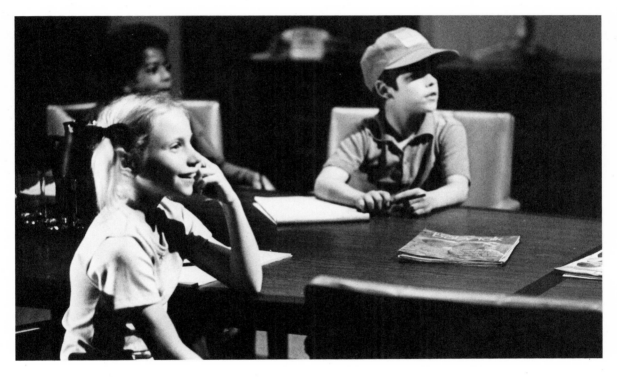

"Well," said Dr. Smith, "the contractions start as a little stomach ache. These are called labor pains, and they do get stronger."

Now Petey was really concerned. "When do they stop?" he asked.

"Petey, this may sound funny, but most women say they don't mind the pain. They know it's well worth it, and it stops the minute the baby is born."

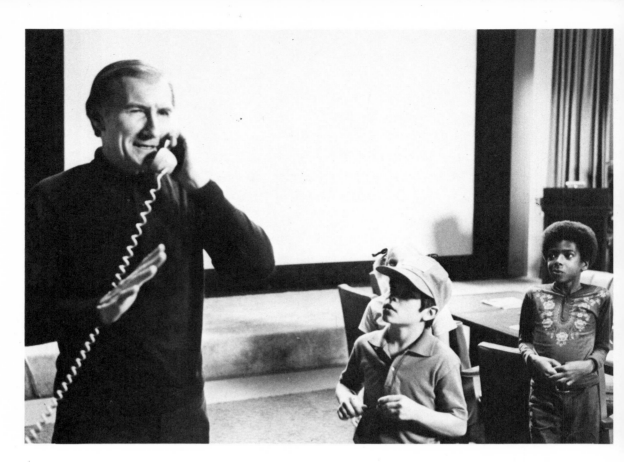

Suddenly, a telephone rang.

"Whoops," said Dr. Smith. "Excuse me." He
pressed a button to turn the lights back on, then walked over
to a desk in the corner of the room. The phone on
the desk rang again and he picked up the receiver.

"Hello, Dr. Smith here," he said. "Oh hello,
Jim." He cupped his hand over the phone and quickly said,
"It's your father, Petey."

Petey ran to Dr. Smith's side.

"I certainly will," Dr. Smith said into the phone.
"Why don't you let him keep me company for a while? We can
wait for the good news together. . . . Great! Give
Anne my love and tell her I'll see you all later. . . . Right.
Bye." He hung up the phone and turned to Petey.

"Petey, your mother's at the hospital!"

Petey looked stunned. Oscar and Kelly crowded
around him.

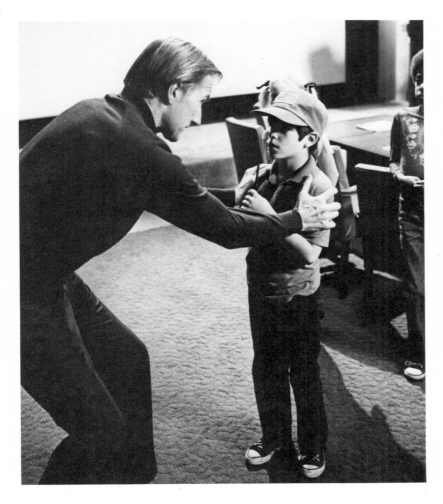

Dr. Smith said, "I told your dad you'd stay
with me in my office until we heard from him. Okay? Oscar
and Kelly, why don't you call your folks and see if
you can stay, too."

"Hey, Petey," Kelly said, "All ri-i-i-ght!!"

"Wahoo!!" Oscar yelled, jumping up and down.

They left the screening room and went into Dr.
Smith's office. The doctor took a bottle of orange juice out of
the refrigerator and lined up some paper cups on the desk.
"This calls for a celebration," he said and poured
juice into each of the cups.

They each reached for a cup, and Dr. Smith raised his in a toast.

"Here's to Petey's mom," he said happily.

"Right!" the children cheered.

Petey grew quiet. "How long before we know?" he said.

"Depends a lot on your little brother or sister," Dr. Smith said. "Some babies are eager; others take their time."

"I hope Mom will be okay," Petey said softly.

"Oh, she'll have the best of care," said Dr. Smith. "Everybody at the hospital will make sure she's comfortable and happy."

For the next hour, the children busied themselves exploring the office. Kelly looked through the microscope. Oscar checked everybody's heartbeat with a stethoscope. Petey paced up and down, like an expectant brother. Dr. Smith did some paper work and answered about a hundred questions.

Petey wanted to know what Dr. Smith thought was happening at the hospital.

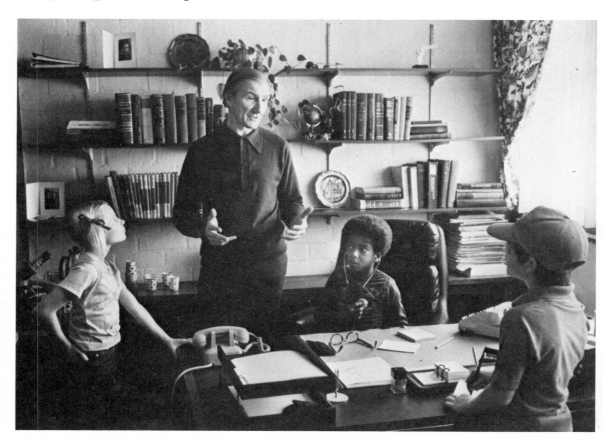

"Well," the doctor said, "when your dad called, the nurses had taken your mom into the labor room. They will stay with her and help her count the contractions. Your dad is with her, too. When the contractions start to get strong and close together, they'll move her into the delivery room. The doctors and nurses will be right there to make sure both your mom and the baby are well cared for."

"They won't leave her alone, will they?" asked Petey.

"Oh, no," said Dr. Smith. "She's the star of the show, the most important person there. They won't leave her, even for a minute."

The phone rang and startled all of them. Petey reached for it, then drew his hand back. Dr. Smith smiled at him and picked up the receiver. Petey, Oscar, and Kelly froze.

"Hello. . . . Oh, Jim, that's wonderful. Congratulations. . . . Yes, of course. . . . Wait, he's right here." The doctor handed the phone to Petey.

"Dad? Hi!" Petey said, excited. "Wow, that's great! . . . Is Mom okay? . . . Oh good. . . Yeah, I'm fine. . . .

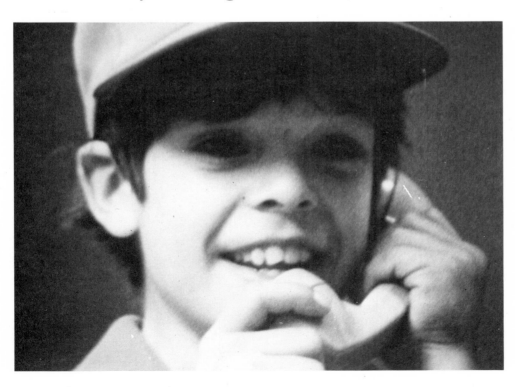

Okay. I'll see you in a little while. Tell Mom I said 'hi'. . . .
Okay, bye." He hung up and grinned. Kelly was clutching
Oscar's arm.

Petey smiled at them. "I've got a baby . . . brother!"
he yelled.

Everybody cheered. Dr. Smith shook Petey's
hand and congratulated him. Kelly and Oscar shrieked
with delight.

Petey's dad took him out to dinner that evening.

"Just think," Mr. Evans said. "We've got a spanking
new baby, Pete!"

"Tell me again what he looks like," Petey said.

"Well, he's about this big," Mr. Evans said, and
gestured with his hands. "And he's got lots of
black hair, and he wrinkles up his whole face. His face
is kind of red, and he's got blue eyes, and he looks just
like . . . guess who?"

"Mom?" Petey asked.

"No."

"You." Petey said.

"Nope." Mr. Evans smiled. "He looks just like YOU!"

"Really?" Petey exclaimed.

"Uh-huh," Mr. Evans said proudly. "Exactly. And
you know what, Pete?"

"What?"

"I hope he grows up to be just like you, 'cause you're
the best son in the whole world."

Petey felt like crying. "Let's go home, Dad," he said.

"Okay, sport. We'll call up Mom and talk to her.

"All right!" Petey said. He really felt good all over.

A few days later, Mrs. Evans and the baby
came home from the hospital. Petey was glad to see his mom,

and she started to cry when she saw him.

"Petey, I missed you so much," she told him.

"Aw, Mom," Petey said.

She sat down on the living-room sofa and unwrapped the bundle in her arms. Petey kneeled down beside her. He peered at the baby and smiled.

"Alex, say hello to your big brother," Mrs. Evans said.

The baby yawned.

Petey grinned. "Hi, Alex," he said. "You sure are funny looking." He gently touched the baby's hand. The baby quickly grabbed his finger and clutched it.

"Look at that!" Petey said. "He really is strong. Boy, what a grip you've got, Alex." He carefully undid the baby's fingers from around his own.

"I'm going to feed him and put him to bed, now," Mrs. Evans said. "He's going to sleep in the bassinette in our room for a few weeks. Then we'll move him into the crib in your room. Okay?"

"Okay," Petey said.

"Come on, Pete," Mr. Evans said. "Let's get lunch ready, while Mom's taking care of the baby. We'll fix our super deluxe grilled-cheese sandwiches."

After lunch, Mrs. Evans took a nap. Mr. Evans told Petey he'd play catch with him, so Petey ran up to his room to get his mitt. He passed his mom's room, and the door was open. He tiptoed into the room and went over to the bassinette. The baby was asleep. Petey looked at him for a long time.

"Alex," he whispered, "When you get bigger, I'm gonna teach you how to play baseball. Nobody's ever been allowed to wear my red hat, but I'm gonna let you wear it. And you can use my mitt, too."

He touched the baby's cheek.

"I'm so glad you're my brother," he said softly.

MY MOM'S HAVING A BABY (song)

Music by Dean Elliott, Lyrics by John Bradford

My mom's having a baby.
That's why she looks that way.
I should be glad
For Mom and Dad.
They want it
Doggone it!
Why should we have a baby?
I can't ask right out loud.
But gee, if three is company
Won't four be a sort of crowd?
My mom's having a baby.

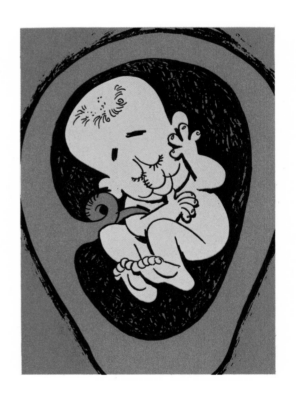